EASING SCIATICA PAIN FOR SENIORS

Effective Exercises to Find Relief and Restore Mobility with Low-Impact Stretches, Core Strengthening Exercises, and Mind-Body Techniques

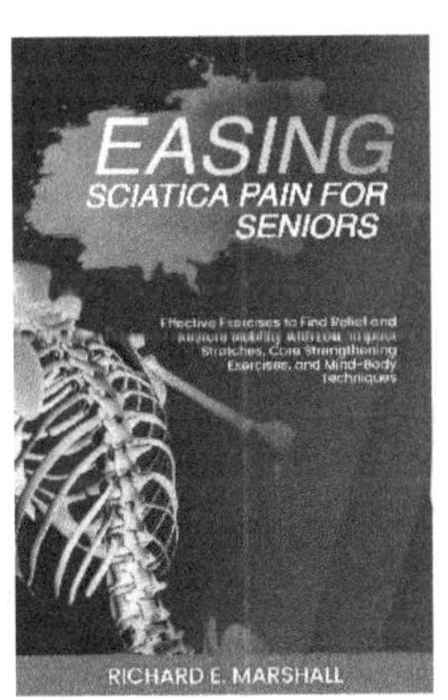

RICHARD E. MARSHALL

GET ACCESS TO MY MORE FITNESS BOOKS

EASING SCIATICA PAIN

INTRODUCTION

The Anatomy of the Sciatic Nerve

Sciatica is lower back discomfort that radiates down the leg. The leg may hurt in front, behind, or on the outside. When engaging in strenuous activity like heavy lifting, onset is frequently abrupt, however it can also happen gradually. It's common to characterize the pain as shooting. Usually, a single side of the body experiences the symptoms. On the other hand, some factors might induce discomfort on both sides. There can occasionally be lower back discomfort. There may be numbness or weakness in different areas of the afflicted foot and leg.

A spinal disc herniation pushing on one of the lumbar or sacral nerve roots is the cause of around 90% of cases of sciatica. Other potential causes of sciatica include pelvic tumors, piriformis syndrome, spondylolisthesis, spinal stenosis, and pregnancy. When diagnosing, the straight-leg-raising test is frequently useful. If the patient feels pain shooting below the knee when their leg is elevated while they are on their back, the test is considered positive.

Medical imaging is usually not required. Imaging, however, could be done if there is a problem with the function of the bowels or bladder, if there is a severe loss of sensation or weakness, if the symptoms are persistent, or if there is a possibility of a tumor or infection. Hip disorders as well as infections like early shingles (before the rash forms) might present similarly. Men have sciatica more often than women, with the condition most commonly affecting those between the ages of 40 and 59. The ailment has been recognized since prehistoric times. The word sciatica was first recorded in usage in 1451.

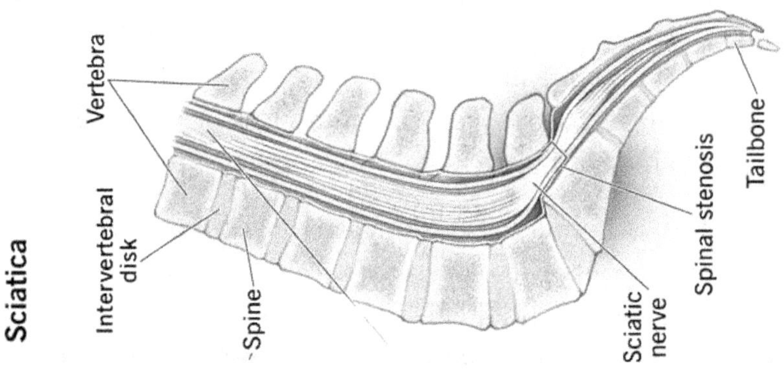

Causes of Sciatica

Sciatica can have many distinct causes, but the most typical one is a herniated disk. When a disk in the spine ruptures or bulges, putting pressure on the sciatic nerve, it is called a herniated disk. This may occur as a result of age, trauma, or abuse.

A damage to the connective tissue and padding between vertebrae, known as a spinal disc herniation, is often brought on by trauma or severe strain on the spine. Physical incapacity, discomfort or feeling in various sections of the body, and back pain are possible outcomes. An MRI is the most reliable diagnosis method for disc herniation, and medications and surgery are possible treatments. Core strength and an understanding of proper body mechanics, especially posture, are the strongest defences against disc herniation.

An intervertebral disc is said to be herniated when a rupture in the outer, fibrous ring causes the soft, middle section to protrude past the damaged outer rings.

Disc herniation is typically brought on by trauma or straining from lifting or twisting, and is often linked to age-related degeneration of the outer ring, or annulus fibrosus. Due to the posterior longitudinal ligament's relative narrowness in comparison to the anterior longitudinal ligament, tears are nearly invariably posterolateral, or on the rear sides. Even in the absence of nerve root compression, a disc ring rip may cause chemicals to be released that cause inflammation and excruciating pain.

Disc herniation is typically the result of an advanced disc protrusion, in which the annulus fibrosis's outermost layers remain intact but may protrude when the disc is compressed. Unlike a herniation, the center does not rupture through the surrounding layers. The majority of mild herniations recover in a few weeks. In general, anti-inflammatory medications work well to relieve pain brought on by disc herniation, protrusion, bulging, or rupture.

Spondylolisthesis is the displacement of one spinal vertebra compared to another. Although spondylolisthesis is described in medical dictionaries as the forward or anterior displacement of a vertebra over the inferior vertebra (or sacrum), it is commonly characterized in textbooks as displacement in any direction. Based on how much one vertebral body slips in relation to the next neighboring vertebral body, spondylolisthesis is graded.

One of the six main causes of spondylolisthesis is categorized as follows: degenerative, traumatic, dysplastic, isthmic, pathologic, or post-surgical. The L5 vertebral body anteriorly translating over the S1 vertebral body is the primary location of spondylolisthesis, which most frequently affects the lumbar spine at the L5-S1 level.

An improper narrowing of the neural foramen or spinal canal that puts pressure on the spinal cord or nerve roots is known as spinal stenosis. Pain, numbness, or weakness in the arms or legs are possible symptoms. Usually, symptoms develop gradually and are better as you lean forward. Loss of control over one's bowels, bladder, or sexual organs are examples of severe symptoms.

Achondroplasia, a hereditary disorder, trauma, rheumatoid arthritis, osteoarthritis, spinal tumors, Paget's disease of the bone, scoliosis, and spondylolisthesis are among the possible causes. Based on the afflicted region of the spine, it may be divided into three categories: lumbar, thoracic, and cervical stenosis. The most prevalent is lumbar stenosis, which is followed by cervical stenosis. Typically, medical imaging and symptoms are used to make a diagnosis.

It is thought that piriformis syndrome is caused by the piriformis muscle compressing the sciatic nerve. The sciatic nerve is the biggest and bulkiest nerve in the human body. It is 2 cm broad and 0.5 cm thick at the origin. The lumbosacral plexus's L4-S3 segments have their origins in the sciatic nerve. The nerve will travel toward the lower limb, passing inferiorly to the piriformis muscle before splitting into the common tibial and fibular nerves. Numbness and soreness in the buttocks and down the leg are possible symptoms. Running or sitting might aggravate symptoms rather often.

Physical Tests

Sciatica may usually be diagnosed if a patient has one leg's typical radiating pain and one or more neurological symptoms of nerve root stress or neurological impairment.

The most common diagnostic test is the straight leg lift to create Lasègue's sign. The test is deemed positive if it reproduces pain in the sciatic nerve distribution when the straight leg is passively flexed between 30 and 70 degrees. Approximately 90% of those with sciatica get a positive result on this test; however, 75% of those who do not have sciatica have a positive result. Sciatica in the afflicted leg may result with straight leg elevation of the unaffected limb; this is referred to as the Fajersztajn sign. Compared to Lasègue's sign, the Fajersztajn sign is a more precise indicator of a herniated disc.

Sciatica pain may become temporarily worse when doing actions that raise intraspinal pressure, such as flexion of the neck, coughing, and bilateral compression of the jugular veins.

Sciatica Risk Factors

Age: People with sciatica are more likely to be between 30 and 60 years old.

Weight: Obesity or being overweight might put more strain on the sciatic nerve.

Occupation: Work involving a lot of lifting, twisting, or bending might raise your chance of developing sciatica.

Smoking: Smoking increases the risk of spinal disk herniation by causing damage to the blood vessels supplying the disks.

Diabetes: Nerves, especially the sciatic nerve, can be harmed by diabetes.

Pregnancy: Because the expanding baby puts extra pressure on the sciatic nerve, pregnant women are more prone to have sciatica.

Benefits of Exercise for Sciatica

Sciatica is a disorder that causes pain to radiate along the sciatic nerve. It may be extremely painful and have a negative impact on a person's quality of life. Even though there are many different ways to treat sciatica pain, a regimented exercise program might be crucial to its successful management. This chapter explores the many advantages of exercise for sciatica, including pain relief, increased flexibility, strengthening of the supporting muscles, decreased inflammation, and accelerated recovery.

Exercise for Sciatica Pain Relief

Pain alleviation is one of the main reasons people with sciatica seek to exercise. By performing certain exercises, the sciatic nerve's compression is lessened, which lessens the severity and frequency of pain episodes. The strain on the nerve decreases as the muscles surrounding the injured area become more flexible and stronger, which significantly lessens sciatic pain.

Increasing Range of Motion and Flexibility

One's range of motion is frequently restricted by stiffness and decreased flexibility caused by sciatica. Reversing these consequences requires exercise, which is crucial. Flexibility can be improved by performing certain stretches and exercises that target the muscles and ligaments around the sciatic nerve. Increased mobility and pain relief are two benefits of increased flexibility that make it easier for people to carry out everyday tasks.

Developing the Spine's Supporting Muscles

Sciatica symptoms may worsen if the muscles supporting the spine are weak. Strengthening the hip, lower back, and core muscles is the main goal of a well-rounded workout program since it gives the spine the support it needs. Strengthening these muscle groups lowers the risk of nerve compression by stabilizing the spine. Targeted workouts like hip-strengthening regimens, back extensions, and core exercises might be included in the category of strengthening exercises.

Exercise-Based Inflammation Reduction

Sciatica is frequently accompanied by inflammation, which exacerbates pain and suffering. It has been demonstrated that exercise has anti-inflammatory properties that aid to lessen the inflammatory response in the injured region. Exercises that increase blood circulation, in particular, help to remove inflammatory byproducts from the body and supply vital nutrients and oxygen to the damaged tissues. Exercise's twin benefits greatly reduce inflammation and the symptoms that go along with it.

Encouraging the Recovery Process

In addition to treating sciatica symptoms, exercise is essential for the recovery process. Exercise helps the body's healing processes by increasing blood flow and oxygenation to the injured area. It enhances general tissue health, lessens the production of scar tissue, and encourages the regeneration of injured tissues. Frequent exercise promotes a more long-lasting and durable outcome for sciatica by helping the body heal from its underlying causes.

Developing a Successful Exercise Program for Sciatica

It is crucial to customize the exercise regimen to each person's demands and limits in order to fully benefit from exercise for sciatica. Getting advice from a trained fitness specialist or a healthcare professional may assist create a customized workout program that targets certain issues and guarantees development that is both safe and efficient.

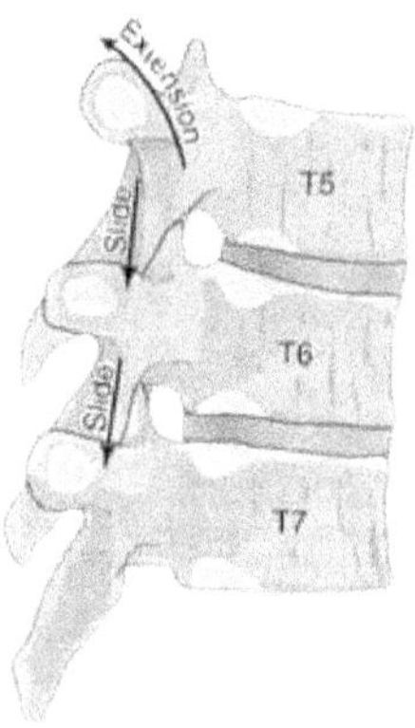

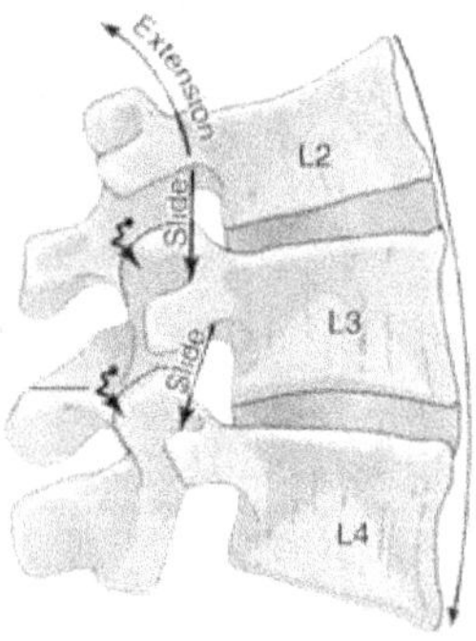

Section I: Exercise Fundamentals

Dynamic Warm-Up Activities

The active warm-up is an essential part of any fitness program, but it's especially important for those with sciatica. It acts as a warm-up, steadily raising body temperature, heart rate, and blood flow while prepping muscles and joints for higher-intensity exercise. A dynamic warm-up for those with sciatica should include increasing range of motion, releasing tense muscles, and making sure the body is ready for the tasks ahead.

Joint mobility exercises: Mild, regulated motions that cover the whole range of motion in joints. This might involve rotating movements of the knees, hips, shoulders, and ankles.

Low-Impact Cardiovascular Exercises: Take part in exercises like elliptical training, stationary cycling, or brisk walking. These movements warm up the muscles and increase blood flow without overstressing the spine.

Dynamic Stretch: Incorporate dynamic stretches that focus on the main muscle groups implicated in sciatica. Dynamic stretches such as leg swings, hip circles, and torso twists can be very helpful.

Exercises for Core Activation: Include poses that gently engage the core muscles, including pelvic tilts, to help stabilize the spine. This is especially important for those who have sciatica since a solid core keeps the lower back from being overworked.

Gradual Intensity Increase: During the warm-up, increase your intensity gradually from low to moderate. By increasing gradually, the body can adjust and the likelihood of exacerbating sciatica symptoms is reduced.

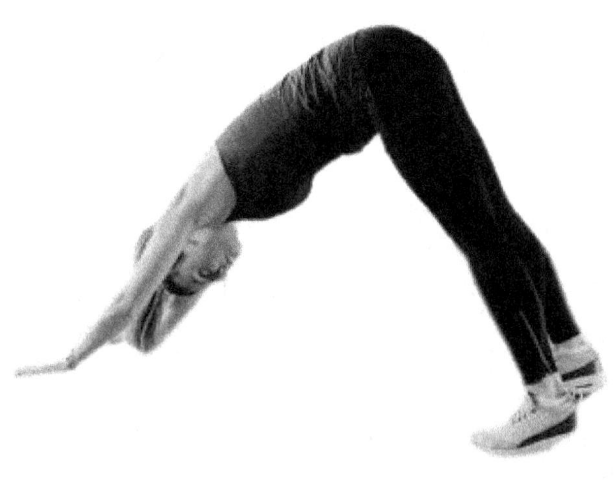

Although it is sometimes overlooked, the cool-down phase is essential for those with sciatica since it increases flexibility, lessens muscular pain, and speeds up recovery. Gentle stretches intended to lengthen muscles, improve flexibility, and aid in a gradual transition back to rest should be the emphasis of cool-down exercises.

Static Stretching: Do stretches that concentrate on the main muscle groups used in the workout. Stretching for the quadriceps, hamstrings, hip flexors, and lower back should be prioritized. Hold each stretch for a duration of 15 to 30 seconds, ensuring a gradual and deliberate release.

Stretch for the Piriformis Muscle: Include a particular stretch for the Piriformis Muscle, considering its importance in sciatica. The sciatic nerve can be effectively relieved of stress by performing the piriformis stretch while seated or lying down.

Balasana, also known as Child's posture, is a gentle yoga posture that stretches the thighs, hips, and lower back. This can be very comforting for people who have sciatica since it releases some of the stress in the lumbar area gently.

Stretch from the Knee to the Chest: While lying on your back, raise one knee toward your chest and hold it there with both hands. This stretch relieves sciatic nerve tension by focusing on the lower back and glutes.

Breathing and Relaxation Exercises: To encourage relaxation and ease any lingering tension, incorporate deep breathing exercises into the cool-down. To activate the parasympathetic nervous system and promote general relaxation, concentrate on diaphragmatic breathing.

Section II: Targeted Exercises

Core Strengthening Exercises

Plank

Target area: muscles in the core, including the abdominals, back, and buttocks.

Steps:

- Start in a push-up position, but instead of lowering yourself down, hold the position for 30-60 seconds.

Reps: 3 sets of 30-60 seconds

Bird Dog

Target area: muscles in the core, as well as the hips and glutes.

Steps:

- With your hands behind your shoulders and your knees beneath your hips, begin on your hands and knees.

- Maintaining a flat back, extend your right arm forward and your left leg back.
- Return to the starting position after three seconds of holding.
- Proceed with the opposite limb and limb.

Reps: 3 sets of 10-12 repetitions per side

Bridge

Target area: muscles in the core, as well as the glutes and hamstrings.

Steps:

- With your feet flat on the ground and your knees bent, lie on your back.
- As you raise your hips off the ground, your shoulders and knees should come in a straight line.
- Lower yourself back to the starting position after three seconds of holding.

Reps: 3 sets of 10-12 repetitions

Crunches

Target area: abdominal area.

Steps:

- With your feet flat on the ground and your knees bent, lie on your back.
- Put your hands crossed over your chest or behind your head.
- Use your abdominal muscles to curl your upper body up towards your knees.
- Return to the starting position slowly.

Reps: 3 sets of 15-20 repetitions

Side Plank

Target area: muscles in the sides of the core, as well as the obliques.

Steps:

- Placing your elbow behind your shoulder and placing your forearm on the ground, lie on your side.
- Form a straight line from your head to your heels by stacking your feet and raising your hips off the floor.
- For 30 to 60 seconds, hold.
- Continue on the opposite side.

Reps: 3 sets of 30-60 seconds per side

NOTE: These exercises can be done 2-3 times per week. It is important to start slowly and gradually increase the intensity of your workouts. You should also listen to your body and stop if you experience any pain.

Stretching for Sciatica Relief

Piriformis Stretch

Target area: piriformis muscle

Steps:

- With your feet flat on the ground and your knees bent, lie on your back.
- Bring your right knee up to your chest by crossing your right ankle over your left knee.
- Till your right buttocks feel stretched, slowly bring your right knee up to your chest.
- After 30 seconds of holding, swap sides.

Reps:3 sets of 30 seconds per side

Knee to Chest Stretch

Target area: hamstrings

Steps:

- With your feet flat on the ground and your knees bent, lie on your back.
- Put your hands around one knee and bring it up to your chest.
- Till the back of your thigh stretches, slowly bring your knee up to your chest.
- After 30 seconds of holding still, return your leg to its initial position.
- Continue with the opposite leg.

Reps: 3 sets of 30 seconds per leg

Seated Spinal Stretch

Target area: elongate the spine

Steps:

- With your legs out in front of you, take a seat on the floor.
- Reaching for your toes, bend forward at the waist.
- Maintain a straight back and a tucked in chin.

- After 30 seconds of holding, carefully go back to the initial position.

Reps: 3 sets of 30 seconds

Lying Knee-to-Chest Stretch

Target area: hip flexors

Steps:

- Stretch your legs out in front of you while lying on your back.
- Put your hands around one knee and bring it up to your chest.
- Till the front of your hip stretches, slowly bring your leg up to your chest.
- After 30 seconds of holding still, return your leg to its initial position.
- Continue with the opposite leg.

Reps: 3 sets of 30 seconds per leg

Lying Hamstring Stretch

Target area: hamstrings

Steps:

- One leg should be straight up in the air while you lie on your back.
- When you feel a stretch in the back of your thigh, slowly bring your leg towards your chest while tying a towel over the ball of your foot.
- After 30 seconds of holding, carefully return your leg to the beginning position.
- Continue with the opposite leg.

Reps: 3 sets of 30 seconds per leg

Standing Hamstring Stretch

Target area: hamstrings

Steps:

- Stand with your feet hip-width apart and place your hands on a wall for support.
- Bend forward at the waist, keeping your back straight and your chin tucked in.
- Reach towards your toes, keeping your legs straight.
- Hold for 30 seconds, then slowly return to the starting position.

Reps: 3 sets of 30 seconds

Standing Quadriceps Stretch

Target area: quadriceps

Steps:

- Position your feet hip-width apart, then bend one knee such that your heel points in the direction of your buttocks.
- Holding onto your ankle, slowly bring your heel up to your buttocks until your front thigh stretches.
- After 30 seconds of holding still, return your leg to its initial position.
- Continue with the opposite leg.

Reps: 3 sets of 30 seconds per leg

Low Back Stretch

Target area: spine

Steps:

- With your toes pointing and your knees hip-width apart, crouch on the ground.
- With your chin tucked in and your back straight, take a seat back on your heels.
- Arms extended aloft, maintain the position for 30 seconds.

- Return to the starting position slowly.

Reps: 3 sets of 30 seconds

NOTE: Please consult your doctor before starting a new stretching routine if you have any concerns.

Low-Impact Cardiovascular Exercises for Sciatica

Walking

Walking is an excellent strategy to increase heart rate and strengthen your cardiovascular system without overstressing your joints. It's also a fairly portable workout that you can perform practically anyplace.

Tips:

- Put on supportive footwear.
- Walk more, further, and more intensely at first, but start off gently.
- If at all feasible, choose a level stroll.
- For further inspiration, go for a walk with a friend or relative.

Swimming

Swimming is a very gentle and low-impact kind of exercise for the joints. It's also a fantastic technique to work out your entire body.

Tips:

- Choose a swimming pool with warm water.
- Take a quick swim to start, then progressively increase the time and intensity of your exercises.
- If you need to, use a flotation device.
- Take breaks when necessary.

Elliptical

The elliptical is a low-impact exercise machine that simulates walking or running without putting stress on your joints.

Tips:

- Your workouts should begin with modest resistance and be gradually increased in intensity.
- For support, hold onto the handles.
- Maintain a straight back and a contracted core.
- If you need to, take breaks.

Stationary Bike

Another low-impact, arthritic-friendly workout is stationary bike riding. It's also a fantastic cardiovascular exercise.

Tips:

- When the pedals are at their lowest position, adjust the seat height so that your legs are slightly bent.
- Your workouts should begin with modest resistance and be gradually increased in intensity.
- Maintain a straight back and a contracted core.
- When necessary, take breaks.

Water Aerobics

One low-impact workout that may be done in a pool is called water aerobics. It's a fantastic approach to strengthen your heart and get a complete body exercise.

Tips:

- Put on some water shoes and a swimsuit.
- Take a water aerobics class that is suitable for your level of fitness to start.
- Pay attention to your body and take pauses as required.

Rowing Machine

Rowing is a low-impact exercise that works the muscles in your arms, legs, and back. It is also a great way to get a cardiovascular workout.

Tips:

- Your workouts should begin slowly and then be intensified progressively.
- Maintain a straight back and a contracted core.
- To assist you keep good form, use the rowing machine's straps.
- When necessary, take breaks.

Stair Climbing

Stair climbing is a great way to get your heart rate up and improve your cardiovascular health. It is also a weight-bearing exercise that can help to strengthen your bones.

Tips:

- Exercise at a leisurely rate at first, then progressively pick up the tempo and intensity.
- For assistance, use the handrails.
- Take breaks when necessary.

Section III: Specialized Workouts

Yoga poses that can help relieve sciatica pain:

Child's Pose (Balasana)

Child's pose is a resting pose that can help to release tension in the lower back and hips. It is also a good pose for stretching the hamstrings.

Steps:

- With your toes together and your knees hip-width apart, crouch on the ground.
- Place your heels back and lean forward so that your forehead rests on the ground or a block.
- Place your arms comfortably beside your body, palms down.
- Take a deep breath and hold it for a few minutes.

Downward-Facing Dog (Adho Mukha Svanasana)

A strengthening position that can assist to increase flexibility in the hamstrings and spine is downward-facing dog. Additionally, it's a great position for opening the shoulders and chest.

Steps:

- With your hands shoulder-width apart and your knees hip-width apart, begin on your hands and knees.
- Form an inverted V shape with your body by tucking your toes under and lifting your hips up and back.
- Maintain a long spine and plant your heels firmly on the ground.
- For five to ten breaths, hold your deep breath.

Pigeon Pose (Kapotasana)

A deep hip-opening stance called pigeon pose can aid in releasing tension in the piriformis muscle, which is frequently implicated in sciatica.

Steps:

- Start on your hands and knees with your hands shoulder-width apart and your knees hip-width apart.
- To align your shin with the front edge of your mat, bend your right knee forward and bring it forward.

- With your right foot flexed, drop your left hip toward the mat.
- Take a deep breath and hold it for 30 to 60 seconds.
- Continue on the opposite side.

Half Lord of the Fishes Pose (Ardha Matsyendrasana)

Half lord of the fishes pose is a twisting pose that can help to release tension in the spine and hips. It is also a good pose for improving digestion and reducing stress.

Steps:

- Seated on the floor, stretch your legs in front of you to begin.
- Your right foot should be outside of your left hip as you cross your body and bend your right knee.
- Turn your upper body to the right and encircle your right knee with your left arm.
- Maintain a long spine while taking deep breaths.
- Hold for a duration of 30 to 1 minute.
- Repeat on the opposite side.

Reclining Bound Angle Pose (Supta Baddha Konasana)

One mild hip-opening position that might help alleviate tension in the hips and lower back is the reclining bound angle stance. It's a beneficial position for both mental and physical relaxation.

Steps:

- Lying on your back, place your feet flat on the floor and bend your knees.
- Your knees should drop to the sides as you bring the soles of your feet together.
- Arms should be relaxed by your sides, palms facing upward.
- For five to ten minutes, hold your deep breath.

Cobbler's Pose (Baddha Konasana)

A deep hip-opening stance that helps alleviate tension in the groin and inner thighs is called Cobbler's pose. Enhancing flexibility in the hips and lower back can also be beneficial.

Steps:

- With your legs out in front of you, take a seat on the floor.

- Let your knees drop to the sides as you bend them and bring the soles of your feet together.
- While bending forward gently, maintain a long spine.
- Raise your arms over your head or lay them across your thighs.
- Take a deep breath and hold it for 30 to 60 seconds.

Bridge Pose (Setu Bandha Sarvangasana)

Bridge pose is a strengthening pose that can help to improve flexibility in the hamstrings, glutes, and lower back. It can also help to open the chest and shoulders.

Steps:

- With your feet hip-width apart and your knees bent, lie flat on your back.
- Put your arms adjacent to your torso with your hands facing down.
- Forming a bridge with your body, press your feet into the floor and raise your hips off the mat.
- Keep your back straight and your thighs parallel to the floor.
- Hold for 10-15 breaths.

Incorporating Yoga in Your Daily Routine

1. Get Started Gradually

If you're new to yoga or sciatica relief, begin with easier postures and work your way up to more challenging ones. Pay attention to your body and try not to push yourself into discomfort.

2. Regularity Is Essential

Try to get in frequent, even 15-minute yoga practices. Maintaining consistency enables your body to adjust and reap the whole rewards of the exercise.

3. Adjust Pose as Necessary

Don't be afraid to adjust positions to suit your comfort level. Yoga is a personal practice, and those with sciatica may find it easier to do with certain modifications.

4. Incorporate meditation and breathwork

Include pranayama, or deep breathing techniques, and meditation in your daily regimen. Enhancing relaxation and lowering stress levels through mindful breathing can help treat sciatica overall.

5. Speak with a Yoga Teacher

If you're new to the practice or have certain health concerns, think about taking a class or speaking with a certified yoga instructor. They are able to guarantee correct alignment and offer tailored coaching.

Pilates Exercises

Pilates exercises for core strength with modifications for sciatica patients:

Pelvic Tilt

This exercise strengthens the deep abdominal muscles that support the spine.

Original Exercise:

- With your feet flat on the ground and your knees bent, lie on your back.
- Gently press your hands on your lower abdomen.
- So that your lower back presses against the floor, tilt your pelvis.
- Hold for three to five seconds, then let go.

Modification for Sciatica:

- Throughout the exercise, keep your feet level on the floor and your knees bent.
- Refrain from slanting your pelvis too much as this may compress your sciatic nerve.

Double Leg Stretch

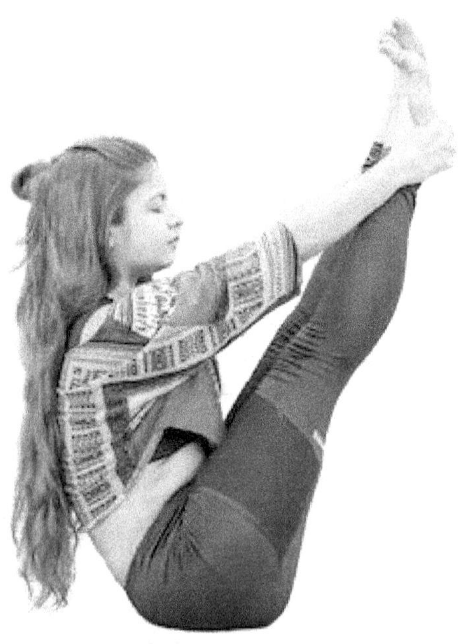

This exercise stretches the hamstrings, which can help to reduce sciatica pain.

Original Exercise:

- With your legs straight up in the air, lie on your back.
- When you feel a stretch in the back of your thighs, gently bring your legs closer to your chest while tying a towel over the balls of your feet.
- After 30 seconds of holding still, carefully return your legs to the beginning position.

Modification for Sciatica:

- Maintain a small bend in your knees the entire time.
- Reducing the distance between your legs and your chest might help relieve sciatica.

Single Leg Stretch

This exercise stretches the hamstrings and quadriceps, which can help to improve flexibility and reduce pain.

Original Exercise:

- With your left leg stretched straight up into the air and your right knee bent, lie on your back.

- When you feel a stretch in the back of your left thigh, slowly bring your left leg towards your chest while tying a towel over the ball of your foot.
- After 30 seconds of holding, carefully return your leg to the beginning position.
- Continue on the opposite side.

Modification for Sciatica:

- Maintain a small bend in your knees the entire time.
- Reducing the distance between your legs and your chest might help relieve sciatica.

Bridge

This exercise strengthens the glutes, hamstrings, and core, which can help to support the spine and reduce sciatica pain.

Original Exercise:

- Lie on your back with your knees bent and your feet flat on the floor.
- Lift your hips off the floor so that your body forms a straight line from your shoulders to your knees.
- Hold for 3-5 seconds and then lower back down to the starting position.

Modification for Sciatica:

- Throughout the exercise, maintain a bent knee position.
- Steer clear of raising your hips excessively since this may compress your sciatic nerve.

Plank

This exercise strengthens the core muscles, which can help to support the spine and reduce sciatica pain.

Original Exercise:

Start in a push-up position, but instead of lowering yourself down, hold the position for 30-60 seconds.

Modification for Sciatica:

- Throughout the exercise, maintain a bent knee position.
- Refrain from maintaining the posture for an extended period of time as this may irritate your sciatic nerve.

Single-Leg Bridge

This exercise can assist to improve stability and lessen sciatica pain by strengthening the core, hamstrings, and glutes on one side at a time.

Original Exercise:

- With your left leg stretched straight up into the air and your right knee bent, lie on your back.
- To make your body create a straight line from your shoulders to your left knee, place your right foot flat on the floor and raise your hips off it.
- Return to the starting position after holding for three to five seconds.
- Continue on the opposite side.

Modification for Sciatica:

- Throughout the exercise, maintain a bent knee position.
- Steer clear of raising your hips excessively since this may compress your sciatic nerve.

Dead Bug

This exercise strengthens the core muscles and improves coordination. It also helps to stretch the hamstrings and lower back.

Original Exercise:

- Stretch your arms straight up toward the sky and your legs straight down toward the floor while lying on your back.
- Elevate your left leg and right arm simultaneously, keeping your back level on the ground.
- Repeat on the other side after lowering your arm and leg back to the beginning position.
- For several repetitions, keep switching between the sides.

Modification for Sciatica:

- Maintain a small bend in your knees the entire time.
- Refrain from raising your legs and arms too high off the ground.

Roll-Up

This exercise strengthens the core muscles and improves flexibility in the spine.

Original Exercise:

- With your feet flat on the ground and your knees bent, lie on your back.
- With your palms facing each other, raise your arms upward.

- As you slowly raise your upper body off the ground, vertebra by vertebra, sit up straight.
- To get back to the initial position, reverse the motion.

Modification for Sciatica:

- Keep your knees bent throughout the exercise.
- Use your arms to support your torso as you curl up.

Double Leg Roll-Up

This exercise strengthens the core muscles and improves flexibility in the spine. It also helps to stretch the hamstrings and lower back.

Original Exercise:

- With your feet flat on the ground and your knees bent, lie on your back.
- Raise your arms straight up and toward the sky.
- As you slowly raise your upper body off the ground, vertebra by vertebra, sit up straight.
- Stretch your legs straight out in front of you as you curl up.
- To get back to the initial position, reverse the motion.

Modification for Sciatica:

- Throughout the exercise, maintain a bent knee position.
- As you curl up, support your torso with your arms.
- Don't spread your legs wide apart.

Scissor Kicks

The hip flexors and core muscles get stronger with this workout. It also aids in enhancing lower back and hip flexibility.

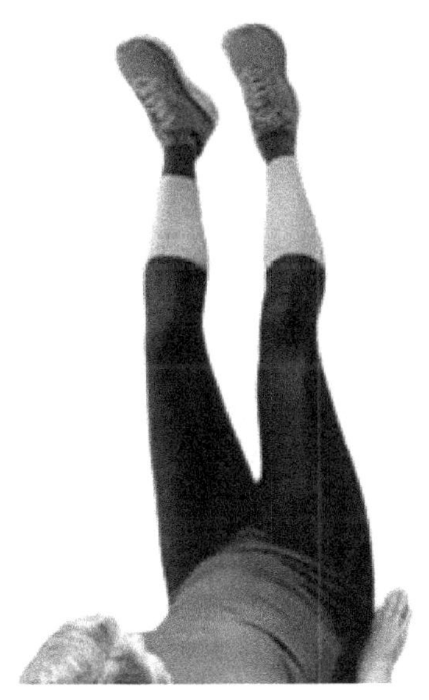

Original Exercise:

- With your legs straight up toward the ceiling and your arms at your sides, lie on your back.
- With your left leg extended and your right leg lowered gradually toward the floor, maintain a flat back on the ground.
- Repeat with your other leg.
- For several repetitions, keep switching between legs.

Modification for Sciatica:

- Maintain a small bend in your knees the entire time.
- Avoid bringing your legs too low to the ground.

Section VI: Lifestyle Modifications

Ergonomics and Daily Habits

Living with sciatica necessitates a multifaceted strategy that goes beyond committed workout programs. The key to reducing symptoms and halting the worsening of sciatic pain is implementing ergonomics and healthy lifestyle choices. Based on real-world experience and professional advice, we explore the significance of appropriate sitting posture, lifting techniques, and sleeping postures in this chapter.

Correct Sitting Posture

Whether it's at a desk, in a car, or while eating, a large amount of the day is spent sitting for many people. Sciatic pain can be exacerbated by bad seating habits. Here's how to keep your sitting posture correct:

Chair and Desk Setup

Tip: Make sure your chair has lumbar support if it's ergonomic. Make sure your workstation is the right height so that, when you rest your elbows on it, they form a 90-degree angle.

Back Support

Tips: To support your lower back's natural arch, place a small cushion or lumbar roll in its curve. This lessens the lumbar spine's strain.

Feet on the Floor

Tips: Make sure your knees are at hip level and keep your feet flat on the ground. Leg crossing should be avoided as it may lead to pelvic misalignment.

Screen Height

Tips: Level up the screen on your computer so that it is at eye level. This keeps the neck from bending too much and encourages a neutral spine.

Frequent Breaks

Tips: Every thirty minutes, take a little pause to stand, stretch, and move about. This encourages circulation and lessens stiffness.

Lifting Methods

Inadequate lifting methods might aggravate sciatic pain and put stress on the lower back. When lifting ordinary or large goods, it's important to use the right techniques:

Bend at the Knees

Tips: bend at the knees but maintain a straight back. Instead of using your back to lift, use your legs and your core muscles.

Keep Things Close

Tips: A helpful hint is to keep the item you're lifting near to your body. As a result, there is less chance of tension on your lower back.

Avoid Twisting

Tips: Instead of twisting your body when you need to turn while holding anything, pivot your feet. Twisting can exacerbate sciatic discomfort and put strain on the lumbar spine.

Use Proper Equipment

To lessen the strain on your back when handling big objects, utilize devices like dollies or carts to spread the weight.

Places to Sleep

Your sleep habits might have a big influence on your sciatica pain. Sleep positions that are appropriate for you can preserve spinal alignment and lessen strain on the sciatic nerve:

Sleeping on Your Back

Tips: Place a cushion beneath your knees if it's comfy for you to do so. This lessens the tension on the lower back and preserves the spine's natural curvature.

Sleeping on Your Side

Tips: To correct your hips and relieve strain on your sciatic nerve and lower back when you sleep on your side, sandwich a pillow between your knees.

Don't Sleep on Your Stomach:

Sleeping on your stomach might cause lower back and neck pain. Make the switch to side or back sleeping, if at all feasible.

High-quality Mattress and Pillows:

Tips: Make an investment in a mattress that keeps your spine in alignment and offers sufficient support. Make use of cushions that accommodate your lower back's and neck's natural curvature.

Anti-Inflammatory Diet

Sciatica and chronic inflammation are frequently linked, which exacerbates pain and suffering. Changing to an anti-inflammatory diet can assist the body's healing process and reduce inflammation. Essential elements of an

Among the anti-inflammatory foods are:

Focus on whole Foods

Tips: Give entire, unprocessed foods first priority. An anti-inflammatory diet is built on nutritious grains, lean meats, and fresh fruits and vegetables.

Omega-3 Fatty Acids

Tips: Include foods high in omega-3 fatty acids, such walnuts, chia seeds, flaxseeds, and fatty fish (mackerel, salmon). These lipids function as anti-inflammatory agents.

Vibrant Fruits and Vegetables

Tips: Eat a range of vibrant fruits and vegetables that are high in phytochemicals and antioxidants. Bell peppers, kale, spinach, and berries are all fantastic options.

Healthy Fats

Tips: opt for good fats such as those found in nuts, avocados, and olive oil. These fats promote general health and have anti-inflammatory properties.

Spices having the Potential to Reduce Inflammation

Tips: Add spices to your food. Examples are garlic, ginger, and turmeric. Certain chemicals found in these spices have anti-inflammatory properties.

Limit Processed Foods

Tips: Reduce your consumption of refined and processed foods because they frequently include trans fats and additives that might aggravate inflammation.

Hydration

Tips: Make sure you're getting enough water to stay hydrated. Drinking enough water promotes all body processes and aids in the removal of pollutants.

Foods that Promote Healthy Nerves

Vitamin B12: The development and operation of nerve cells depend on vitamin B12. Meat, poultry, fish, eggs, and fortified dairy products are good sources of vitamin B12.

Vitamin B6: Vitamin B6 is involved in both pain management and nerve regeneration. B6-rich foods include potatoes, chickpeas, bananas, and chicken.

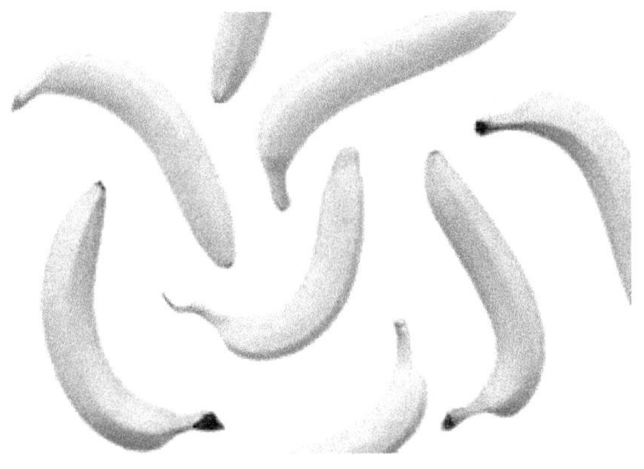

Vitamin D: Vitamin D helps to develop and repair nerves. Good sources of vitamin D include fortified dairy products, fatty fish, and egg yolks.

Magnesium: Magnesium has a role in both muscle relaxation and nerve signal transmission. Rich sources of magnesium include whole grains, nuts, seeds, and leafy greens.

Protein for Muscle Health: Maintaining muscle mass requires consuming enough protein. Incorporate into your diet sources of lean protein such as fish, chicken, beans, and tofu.

Healthy Carbohydrates: Expert Advice: Go for complex carbs like those found in fruits, vegetables, and whole grains. They promote general health and offer long-lasting vitality.

Foods High in Antioxidants: Experience Advice: Antioxidants aid in preventing harm to many types of cells, including nerve cells. A range of fruits and vegetables should be included, particularly those high in vitamins A, C, and E.

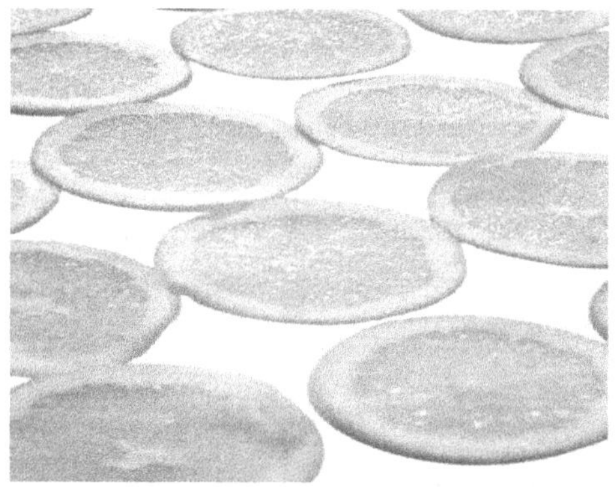

Section V: Progression and Maintenance

How to Effectively Manage Sciatica by Tracking and Modifying Your Exercise Program

A comprehensive strategy that includes both medical intervention and lifestyle adjustments is needed to properly manage sciatica. Exercise is essential for lowering discomfort, increasing flexibility, and strengthening the muscles that support the spine. However, in order to prevent exacerbating your sciatica symptoms, it is imperative that you closely monitor your workout regimen and make any adjustments.

1. Tracking Growth

Effective therapy of sciatica requires keeping a thorough journal of your workout regimen and advancement. You may adjust your program by keeping note of the exercises you perform and determining which ones help or exacerbate your symptoms. Observe elements such as:

- length and level of intensity during workouts
- certain exercises carried out

- Pain intensity prior to, during, and following exercise Any changes to range of motion or flexibility

NOTE: Examine your progress diary on a regular basis to spot trends and modify your workout regimen as necessary.

2. Identifying Danger Signals

While sciatica sufferers might benefit from exercising, it's important to detect any warning symptoms that might mean you need to adjust your regimen or consult a doctor. These red flags consist of:

- increased discomfort or pain during or after physical activity
- tingling or numbness in the afflicted limb
- weakness or lack of coordination in the afflicted limb
- Pain that travels from the buttocks to the foot, either new or worsening

3. Including Mind-Body Methods

When combined with conventional physical exercises, mind-body methods can greatly improve sciatica therapy.

These methods, which include body awareness, flexibility, and relaxation, can help with pain management and general well-being. Examples of these methods include yoga, Pilates, and tai chi.

Yoga: For sciatica sufferers, yoga positions that target the lower back, hips, and hamstrings can be very helpful.

Pilates: The core muscles are the focus of Pilates exercises, which are important for stabilizing the spine and easing sciatic nerve discomfort.

Tai Chi: This mild form of exercise that emphasizes balance and coordination can help with hip and lower back discomfort by increasing flexibility.

4. Relaxation and Stress Reduction

Stress can make sciatica symptoms worse by raising inflammation and stress in the muscles. Including stress-reduction methods in your daily routine can aid with pain management and enhance general wellbeing. Techniques for reducing stress that work well include:

Deep breathing exercises: Pranayama, also known as diaphragmatic breathing, helps ease tension in the muscles and assist relax the nervous system.

Meditation: Practicing mindfulness meditation can assist develop inner calm and ease tension brought on by stress.

Progressive muscle relaxation: This method promotes relaxation and lessens discomfort by tensing and relaxing various muscle groups throughout the body.

5. Meditation and Mindfulness

Meditation and other mindfulness techniques can be very helpful in managing sciatica because they increase bodily awareness, lower stress levels, and encourage relaxation. Mindfulness is a technique that helps reduce pain and enhance general wellbeing by focusing on the present moment and accepting pain sensations without passing judgment.

Living Well with Sciatica

a state that necessitates tolerance, flexibility, and self-care dedication. Sciatica, or pain radiating down the sciatic nerve, can cause severe impairments, impairing movement and interfering with day-to-day activities. However, sciatica may be efficiently managed and a fulfilling life can be had with the appropriate treatment and a positive outlook.

1. Accepting Patience: Moving at a Calm and Slow Speed

Adapting to sciatica necessitates a profound mental change. The days of putting up with agony and waiting for instant relief are long gone. Rather, the key is to exercise patience and take a methodical and gradual approach. This entails paying attention to your body, taking pauses when required, and gradually changing your way of life.

2. Adaptability: Being Adjustable and Willing to Change

Sciatica can throw curveballs at you unexpectedly, so you need to be flexible and willing to change. Enjoyable activities might need to be changed or put on hold for a while. This might entail switching from high-impact to low-impact exercise regimens, figuring out new walking routes each day, or rearranging your workspace.

3. Self-Care: Making wellbeing a priority

Taking care of oneself is crucial while dealing with sciatica. This includes mental, emotional, and physical health. Give priority to things that will benefit your body, such consistent exercise, a healthy diet, and enough sleep. Take up relaxing and enjoyable hobbies, such as reading, listening to music, or going on a nature walk.

4. Mind-Body Link: Developing Inner Power

In order to effectively manage sciatica, the mind-body link is essential. While mindfulness and relaxation can aid in the healing process, stress and worry can make pain worse. To develop inner strength and resilience, try yoga, meditation, or deep breathing exercises.

5. Seeking Assistance: Establishing a Care Team

Consult with medical doctors, physical therapists, and pain management specialists without holding back. Their knowledge and direction can be very helpful in creating a customized treatment plan and successfully treating your sciatica.

6. Knowledge and Self-Determination: Recognizing Your Body

Learn as much as you can about sciatica, including its causes and possible treatments. With this information, you will be able to advocate for your own well-being and make well-informed decisions regarding your treatment.

7. Honoring Minor Wins: Recognizing Development

Although managing sciatica might be difficult, it's important to acknowledge and appreciate little accomplishments along the road. Recognize and value any reduction in your degree of discomfort, degree of flexibility, or general state of health. These tiny triumphs act as progress markers and sources of motivation.

8. Adopting a Holistic Perspective: Tackle the Fundamental Cause

As important as symptom management is, treating the underlying causes of sciatica should not be overlooked. This might entail controlling weight, strengthening the core muscles, or correcting postural abnormalities. You can lessen the possibility of recurrent pain episodes by treating the underlying reasons.

9. Discovering Joy in Motion: Revisiting Movement

Sciatica can make moving uncomfortable, but it's crucial to rediscover the enjoyment of movement. Examine low-impact activities such as yoga, strolling, or swimming. These exercises can increase muscular strength, increase flexibility, and enhance general wellbeing.

10. Living a Meaningful Life: A Self-Discovery Journey

Being sciatica-affected requires self-discovery. It's about adjusting your lifestyle, learning to listen to your body, and putting your health first. You are capable of efficiently managing your sciatica and leading a satisfying life if you have self-care, flexibility, and patience.